Home Care Heart Care

"Building A Legacy of Compassion"

By

Dr. Maria Santiago

Home Care Heart Care

"Building A Legacy of Compassion"

Published by Corner Stone International Enterprises Inc.

978-1-967875-02-3

DEDICATION

This book is dedicated to:

The caregivers, nurses, home health aides, and healthcare professionals who dedicate their lives to providing comfort, dignity, and healing.

To the families who entrust their loved ones to the care of compassionate hands.

To the visionaries, advocates, and leaders who tirelessly work to transform healthcare and ensure that compassion remains at its core.

And to my unwavering supporters, colleagues, mentors, friends, and loved ones who have inspired and strengthened my commitment to building a better future in home healthcare.

This book is a tribute to your dedication, resilience, and the immeasurable impact you make in the lives of others.

With deep gratitude,

Dr. Maria Santiago

Table of Contents

Foreword: A Message to All Disciples of Healthcare

To those who have answered the sacred call to serve, heal, and uplift, this message is for you.

Healthcare is more than a profession; it is a mission, a lifelong commitment to compassion, excellence, and advocacy. Whether you are a caregiver, a nurse, a physician, a home health aide, or a leader shaping policies that define the future of care, you are part of a movement far greater than yourself. You are a disciple of healing, a guardian of dignity, and a voice for those who rely on your knowledge, your skill, and most importantly, your heart.

I have dedicated my life to advancing healthcare education and ensuring that every individual in this field is equipped not only with technical expertise but with an unwavering dedication to those they serve. Through the Home Health Aide Training Institute and my work across national and global platforms, I have seen firsthand how compassionate care transforms lives. Healthcare is not simply about procedures and treatments, it is about presence, about ensuring that no patient, no elderly person, no vulnerable life is ever forgotten or left without dignity.

As disciples of healthcare, you have the power to change the world, one patient, one family, one community at a time. Hold fast to the values that brought you here. Embrace the challenges as opportunities for growth. Lead with empathy, with wisdom, and with the understanding that true healing begins in the heart.

Together, let us build a legacy, one founded on care, compassion, and the unwavering pursuit of excellence.

Dr. Maria Santiago

Introduction

Compassion lies at the heart of every great healthcare endeavor. Home care, in particular, is not just about providing medical assistance, it is about creating a support system that allows individuals to thrive in the comfort of their homes, surrounded by dignity, respect, and care. As the founder of the Home Health Aide Training Institute, I have witnessed firsthand how a well-trained, compassionate caregiver can transform lives, not just for the patients they serve but for entire families and communities.

Throughout my journey, I have worked to ensure that home health professionals are equipped with the knowledge, skills, and empathy necessary to provide exceptional care. I have seen the intersection of healthcare and advocacy and how leadership in this space can shape policies that improve lives. But beyond the institutions and formal training, there is a human element that must never be lost, a commitment to care that extends beyond duty and responsibility and embraces healing with the heart.

This book is a reflection of those values. It is for the caregivers who wake up every day determined to make a difference. It is for the families searching for the right support and guidance. It is for healthcare leaders looking to enhance the field of home care and establish lasting change. Through real-life experiences, insights from my work on national and global boards, and the lessons I've learned in merging healthcare and media, "Home Care, Heart Care" serves as both a guide and a tribute to those who dedicate themselves to compassionate service.

As you read these pages, I invite you to explore the essence of home care, the impact of advocacy, and the power of compassion in shaping a legacy, one that ensures every patient receives the care, respect, and dignity they deserve.

Dr. Maria Santiago

Chapter One: The Heart of Home Care

Home care is more than a service, it is a lifeline, an act of compassion that nurtures both the body and spirit. It is the unseen force that allows individuals to age with dignity, heal in familiar surroundings, and feel the warmth of human connection when they need it most. At its core, home health care is about trust, respect, and the unwavering belief that every person deserves care tailored to their unique needs.

I have witnessed firsthand the profound impact that home health aides, nurses, and caregivers have on the lives they touch. These professionals are not just providers; they are protectors, listeners, advocates, and sometimes, the only consistent presence in a patient's life. Their work is deeply personal, requiring not only skill but a heart willingness to serve.

When I founded the Home Health Aide Training Institute, my vision was to create more than a program, it was to build a movement, a foundation where caregivers would be empowered with knowledge and inspired by purpose. I knew that the demand for quality home care was increasing, yet the standards needed to rise alongside it. It was not enough to teach techniques and procedures; true caregivers needed to understand the *why* behind their work, the human element that turns care into healing.

One of the greatest lessons I have learned in this field is that home care is not just about medical assistance. It is about presence. Sitting beside an elderly patient who has lost their spouse. Holding the hand of someone struggling with a terminal diagnosis. Listening to the stories that no one else has the patience to hear. These moments shape the caregiver's journey as much as they shape the lives of the patients they serve.

But this profession is not without challenges. Caregivers often work long hours with little recognition, pouring their energy into others while navigating emotional exhaustion. The weight of responsibility can be overwhelming, and yet, they continue. Not because they must, but because they "believe" in the power of care.

As we look toward the future, we must ask: How do we continue to honor the heart of home care? How do we ensure that caregivers receive the support, respect, and resources they need to sustain their work? It begins with education, advocacy, and an unwavering commitment to elevating the standard of care.

Through this book, I invite you to reflect on the essence of home healthcare, not just as a profession, but as a calling. Whether you are a caregiver, a family member seeking support, or a leader shaping policy, you hold a place in this journey. Together, we build more than a service, we build a legacy of compassion, one life at a time.

Chapter Two: Founding The Movement

Every great transformation begins with a vision, a deep, unwavering belief that something can and must be better. For me, that vision was rooted in the fundamental need for high-quality, compassionate home healthcare. When I founded the Home Health Aide Training Institute, I wasn't just establishing another program; I was launching a movement, one that would elevate the standards of care and empower those who provide it.

Home healthcare has long been the backbone of support for individuals who wish to remain in their homes rather than transitioning to medical facilities. Yet, despite its critical role, the field has often been overlooked, underfunded, and undervalued. Caregivers, those on the front lines of this work, have frequently been undertrained, underappreciated, and overburdened. I knew that had to change.

The journey of founding the institute was not without its challenges. There were financial obstacles, industry skepticism, and the need to convince others that training home health aides went far beyond teaching routine care, it required instilling compassion, professionalism, and a deep understanding of the human experience. But I was determined. I had seen firsthand how proper training could transform not only the lives of caregivers but also the well-being of the individuals they served.

The foundation of this movement was simple: "education, empowerment, and advocacy." Home health aides are more than service providers; they are lifelines, trusted companions, and protectors of dignity. By creating a program that emphasized both technical skills and the heart of caregiving, I wanted to ensure that every patient, regardless of age, condition, or economic status, received care that was meaningful and life-affirming.

From the beginning, the institute was built to break barriers. It welcomed individuals from diverse backgrounds, trained them rigorously, and equipped them with not only medical knowledge but the emotional intelligence to handle the complexities of caregiving. It didn't take long before the impact became evident. Graduates of the program were not just securing jobs; they were leading change. They were bringing dignity back into healthcare, supporting families in crisis, and proving that caregiving is one of the most honorable professions in the world.

But founding this movement was only the beginning. The future of home healthcare depends on continued advocacy, innovation, and leadership.

This is not just about creating caregivers, it's about cultivating "change agents" who will push for better policies, stronger protections, and a deeper respect for the work that keeps communities thriving.

"Home Care, Heart Care" is not just a title; it is a commitment, one that started with a vision and continues to expand through every caregiver trained, every life touched, and every family supported. This movement is a promise to never let home healthcare fade into the background but to bring it forward as an essential, respected, and empowered profession.

This journey is far from over, and it is one I invite you to take with me.

Chapter Three: The Role of Compassion in Healthcare

Compassion is the silent force that transforms healthcare from a system into a sanctuary. It is the difference between clinical service and human connection, between treating a condition and healing a person.

For too long, healthcare has been measured in numbers: the efficiency of treatment, the speed of diagnosis, the financial cost of care. But behind every statistic is a person, a family, a story, a moment where kindness can mean the difference between hope and despair.

Compassion is not just a virtue in healthcare; it is a necessity. It empowers caregivers to see beyond charts and symptoms, to recognize fear in a patient's eyes, and to extend a hand when words fail. It is the foundation of trust, the bridge between patient and provider, and the reason healthcare must always be anchored in humanity.

Compassion in Practice

In home healthcare, where caregivers step into the intimate spaces of patients' lives, compassion is even more vital. A home health aide is not just a professional; they become part of the fabric of a patient's daily routine. They are the ones who listen to stories long forgotten, who notice the subtle changes in a patient's mood, who understand when silence speaks louder than words.

Compassion is seen in small but powerful ways, a caregiver adjusting their schedule to accommodate a patient's emotional needs, a nurse taking the extra time to explain a treatment plan, a doctor choosing reassurance over rushed efficiency. These moments may never be documented, but their impact is immeasurable.

The Science of Compassion

Studies show that compassion leads to better patient outcomes, faster recovery, increased adherence to treatment, and overall improved mental well-being. Patients who feel heard and respected are more likely to trust their caregivers, and trust is a key ingredient in healing.

But compassion benefits caregivers, too. When healthcare professionals approach their work with empathy, they find greater meaning in their roles, reducing burnout and increasing fulfillment. Compassion is not a drain; it is a source of renewal.

Compassion as a Legacy

As leaders, advocates, and caregivers, we must ensure that compassion is embedded in the future of healthcare. It must be taught, encouraged, and recognized as the foundation of great care. Whether through policy changes, caregiver education, or simple acts of kindness, we must commit to making healthcare not only effective but profoundly human.

Because at the end of the day, medicine treats the body, but compassion heals the soul.

Chapter Four: Leadership in Healthcare Advocacy

Leadership in healthcare is more than decision-making and policy implementation, it is a commitment to championing the rights, dignity, and well-being of individuals who rely on the system for care. Healthcare advocacy requires boldness, resilience, and the ability to navigate both challenges and opportunities to create meaningful, lasting change.

At the heart of healthcare advocacy is the understanding that access to quality care should not be a privilege, but a fundamental right. Whether advocating for better home health standards, policy reform, or increased support for caregivers, true leaders in this space recognize that their role extends beyond administration, it is about impact.

The Role of Leadership in Driving Change

Healthcare leaders, whether running institutions, sitting on advisory boards, or mentoring future professionals, serve as the voice for those who may otherwise go unheard. Advocacy in healthcare requires speaking up for the needs of patients, ensuring that underserved communities receive adequate support, and pushing for policies that improve standards of care.

I have had the honor of serving on national and global boards, collaborating with policymakers, and shaping initiatives that address the evolving needs of healthcare professionals and patients alike. Through these experiences, I've learned that leadership is not just about authority, it is about influence, responsibility, and the ability to inspire action.

Building Bridges Between Healthcare and Policy

One of the greatest challenges in healthcare advocacy is bridging the gap between care providers and policymakers. Often, those making legislative decisions are removed from the day-to-day realities of patients and caregivers. As leaders, we must work to ensure that healthcare reforms are informed by real-world experiences and guided by the voices of those who deliver and receive care.

Advocacy involves engaging with government agencies, nonprofit organizations, and thought leaders to develop strategies that advance healthcare equity, funding, and education. In the realm of home healthcare, this means advocating for fair wages for caregivers, ensuring proper certification standards, and expanding resources for aging populations and vulnerable individuals.

The Intersection of Healthcare and Media

Healthcare advocacy is no longer confined to boardrooms and policy meetings, it has expanded into public discourse, media platforms, and storytelling. As host of "Talk with Maria", I have witnessed firsthand how media can be a powerful tool in shaping public perception and mobilizing support for healthcare initiatives. When leveraged effectively, storytelling in entertainment and journalism can amplify the voices of caregivers, patients, and experts, bringing attention to critical healthcare issues in ways that traditional advocacy sometimes cannot.

Legacy Through Leadership

To be a leader in healthcare advocacy is to build a legacy that extends beyond personal achievements. It is about leaving behind a system that is stronger, more equitable, and more compassionate than it was before. True leadership is measured not by titles, but by the impact one has on individuals, communities, and the future of healthcare.

As we move forward, the call to lead remains ever-present. Whether as a caregiver, a policymaker, a mentor, or an advocate, each of us holds the power to influence healthcare for the better. The question is, how will we use that power?

Chapter 5: Merging Healthcare with Media

Healthcare and media may seem like two entirely different worlds, one rooted in science, policy, and patient care, the other driven by storytelling, entertainment, and influence. Yet, in today's interconnected landscape, media has become one of the most powerful tools for shaping public perception, advocating for change, and bringing critical healthcare issues to the forefront.

For years, healthcare has relied on traditional methods of education and outreach, medical journals, policy debates, and institutional reports. While these remain valuable, they often fail to reach the broader public in ways that truly engage, inspire, and mobilize action. This is where the media steps in, transforming healthcare advocacy from a specialized conversation into a global movement.

The Power of Storytelling in Healthcare

One of the most effective ways to humanize healthcare issues is through storytelling. Data and statistics may inform, but stories move people to act. A well-crafted documentary, a compelling interview, or even a personal testimony shared through digital platforms can make healthcare struggles tangible and relatable. Whether highlighting the life of a caregiver, exploring the challenges of home healthcare, or shedding light on disparities in medical access, media has the unique ability to turn clinical narratives into stories of resilience, hope, and change.

As host of "Talk with Maria," I have witnessed firsthand how conversations about healthcare can spark new perspectives, change misconceptions, and amplify the voices of those on the front lines. When leaders, caregivers, and advocates come together to discuss their experiences in an accessible format, the public engages with healthcare in a way that goes beyond policy discussions, it becomes personal.

Leveraging Entertainment for Advocacy

Entertainment has long been a vehicle for social change. Films, television series, and digital media can introduce audiences to real healthcare issues, sparking conversations and encouraging reforms. Consider how medical dramas shape public understanding of the healthcare profession, how news segments influence policy discussions, and how influential figures use their platforms to advocate for health initiatives.

Healthcare professionals and organizations must embrace the media as an essential part of advocacy, working alongside creators, journalists, and influencers to ensure that accurate, impactful narratives reach the public. Whether through television, podcasts, social media campaigns, or interactive digital platforms, healthcare and media must work together to inform, educate, and inspire action.

Building a Healthcare Media Strategy

For leaders and advocates in healthcare, merging the two industries requires strategic communication. The key is understanding how to craft messages that resonate, engage, and drive meaningful change. Media platforms must be used not just to inform but to connect, turning healthcare discussions into movements that encourage awareness, policy reform, and better patient care.

Healthcare organizations should consider:

- Collaborating with media professionals to create accessible and compelling health-related content.

- Using digital platforms to share patient and caregiver stories.

- Partnering with entertainment influencers to promote health campaigns.

- Developing community-driven media projects that highlight pressing healthcare needs.

A Unified Future for Healthcare and Media

The future of healthcare depends not only on medical advancements but also on how well we communicate those advancements to the world. By embracing media as a tool for advocacy, education, and engagement, we can create a healthcare system that is not only efficient but emotionally connected to those it serves.

Healthcare is a story, one of compassion, challenge, innovation, and resilience. It is time we tell that story in a way that reaches every home, every community, and every nation.

Chapter 6: The Future of Home Health Care

The world is changing, and with it, the way we care for the most vulnerable among us. As medical advancements accelerate, populations age, and healthcare systems face mounting pressures, home health care stands at the forefront of a new era, one that prioritizes personalized, compassionate, and accessible care for all.

In recent years, home health care has evolved beyond its traditional role of assisting the elderly or chronically ill. It has become a critical pillar of modern medicine, enabling individuals to receive quality care without the disruption and expense of institutional settings. But where does it go from here?

Innovation and Technology in Home Care

The future of home health care will be shaped by "technology". Remote patient monitoring, telemedicine, and AI-driven diagnostics are already transforming the way care is delivered. Wearable devices can track vitals in real time, smart medication dispensers ensure adherence to prescriptions, and virtual consultations allow patients to receive expert guidance without leaving their homes.

Artificial intelligence will further optimize care by predicting potential health risks, customizing treatment plans, and streamlining administrative processes for caregivers. The fusion of technology and compassion will allow healthcare professionals to focus less on logistics and more on human connection.

The Growing Demand for Home Care Professionals

As life expectancy rises, the need for skilled home health aides, nurses, and caregivers will continue to grow. The future of home care depends on strong "education and workforce development" ensuring that caregivers are well-trained, fairly compensated, and supported in their careers.

Institutions must invest in caregiver training programs that go beyond the basics, emphasizing holistic care, mental health awareness, and specialized skillsets to serve diverse populations. Governments and organizations must push for better policies that protect the rights and wages of caregivers, making home health care a respected and sustainable profession.

Personalized, Patient-Centric Care

Healthcare is moving away from one-size-fits-all treatments and embracing "personalized medicine". Home health care must follow this trend, adapting services to fit the unique needs of each patient. Cultural sensitivity, customized wellness plans, and an emphasis on emotional well-being will play a greater role in determining how care is provided.

Expanding Access to Home Care

Equity remains a key challenge. While home healthcare has become more mainstream, many communities, especially those in rural or underserved areas, still struggle with access. Advocacy efforts must focus on expanding home care services to ensure that income, geography, and background do not determine the quality of care a person receives.

Investments in mobile healthcare units, digital consultations, and policy reforms will be essential in closing this gap. Home health care must become a standard option, not a privilege reserved for those who can afford it.

A Legacy of Compassion

As the landscape of healthcare shifts, one thing must remain unchanged: "compassion." No matter how advanced technology becomes, no matter how many reforms are passed, home care will always be built on human connection. The future of home healthcare is not just about efficiency, it is about preserving dignity, ensuring comfort, and honoring the humanity of those who rely on it.

We stand at a crossroads where innovation, advocacy, and heart must come together to shape the next chapter of care. Home healthcare is not just adapting to the future, it is "leading it."

Conclusion

Compassion is the foundation of home healthcare, shaping the way we serve, advocate, and innovate. The journey outlined in this book, through leadership, advocacy, and the merging of healthcare with media, underscores the importance of treating home care not just as a profession but as a movement.

The future of home healthcare depends on those willing to push boundaries, challenge outdated systems, and ensure every patient receives care that preserves dignity and enhances quality of life. From the caregiver offering emotional support to the policymaker fighting for reform, we all have a role in shaping what comes next.

Let this book serve as a call to action. Whether you are a caregiver, a healthcare leader, or simply someone invested in improving the lives of others, know that your work matters. Home care is more than a service, it is a legacy of compassion.

May we continue to lead with empathy, advocate with purpose, and always remember that the heart of healthcare lies in the humanity we bring to it.

A Special Message from Dr. Maria Santiago to Apostle Asia Francis & Corner Stone International Enterprises Inc.

To the incredible Apostle Asia Francis, and the dedicated publishing team at Corner Stone International Enterprises,

With a heart full of gratitude, I extend my deepest appreciation for your unwavering support, encouragement, and commitment to bringing Home Care, Heart Care: Building a Legacy of Compassion to life. From the very beginning, your vision, expertise, and dedication have been instrumental in ensuring that this book reaches those who need it most.

Publishing is more than just producing a book, it is about creating a platform for impact, for education, and for transformation. Your belief in this project, coupled with the resources and guidance you have provided, has turned this vision into a reality. Your partnership has made this journey not only possible but deeply rewarding.

Apostle Asia Francis, your leadership, faith, and passion for empowering others serve as an inspiration. Your commitment to excellence and service aligns perfectly with the heart of this book: compassion, advocacy, and lasting change. To the Corner Stone International Enterprises team, your dedication to quality, integrity, and purpose-driven publishing is evident in every step of this process.

This book is not just my work, it is "our shared mission". It is a reflection of the collective effort, faith, and determination that make meaningful work possible. My hope is that it will touch lives, inspire caregivers, and ignite conversations that shape the future of home healthcare.

Thank you for standing alongside me on this journey, for believing in this message, and for ensuring that its impact reaches far and wide. May our work together continue to uplift, educate, and transform lives for generations to come.

With heartfelt appreciation,
Dr. Maria Santiago

About the Author

Dr. Maria Santiago is a visionary leader, healthcare advocate, and media personality dedicated to transforming the landscape of home healthcare and beyond. As the founder of the Home Health Aide Training Institute, a nonprofit committed to equipping caregivers with the knowledge and compassion needed to provide exceptional home health services, she has been instrumental in shaping the future of caregiving.

With a deep passion for both healthcare and entertainment, Dr. Santiago merges her expertise to educate, inspire, and advocate for policy reforms that elevate the standards of care. She serves on numerous national and global boards, using her influence to drive meaningful change in healthcare access, caregiver support, and patient dignity.

Dr. Santiago is also the host of "Talk with Maria", a dynamic talk show where she engages with experts, thought leaders, and change makers to spark conversations that matter. Through her platform, she amplifies voices in healthcare, business, and advocacy, bridging the gap between service and storytelling.

With her unwavering dedication to improving lives, "Home Care, Heart Care: Building a Legacy of Compassion" is not just a book; it is an extension of Dr. Santiago's mission to ensure that caregiving remains rooted in empathy, excellence, and purpose.

www.ingramcontent.com/pod-product-compliance
Lightning Source LLC
Chambersburg PA
CBHW071348290326
41933CB00041B/3109